Hey Doc This is My Story

A Guided Journal & Gift: Share the Heart Behind Your Story

Hope Fields

1957 Publishing

My Record Page...

Full Name: ____

Preferred Name: ____

Gender: __________________ Date of Birth: ____/____/______

Height: _______ Weight:________ Blood Type: ______________

Known Allergies: _______________________________________

____

Medical Conditions to Note: _____________________________

____

____

____

Medications to Avoid: ___________________________________

____

Emergency Contact Name: _________________________________

Number: _______________ Relationship: ____________________

____

Primary Care Doctor: ____________________________________

____

Main Specialist/s: _______________________________________

____

____

____

Health Background Page...

Diagnoses: ______________________________

____

____

____

____

____

____

____

(e.g., Breast Cancer Stage 3, Rheumatoid Arthritis, Anxiety Disorder)

Major Surgeries & Dates: ______________________________

____

____

Current Medications & Dosage: ______________________________

____

____

Suppliments & Herbal Remedies: ______________________________

____

____

Things that don't work for me: ______________________________

____

____

Interior design, and guided prompt format by Hope Fields.
Published by 1957 Publishing.

Hey Doc, This Is My Story
A Guided Journal from the "Guided Journals with Hope" Series
Written by Hope Fields

Preface

The Day I stopped sugar-coating my answers to sugar-coated questions

THERE ARE MOMENTS IN life that brand themselves into memory – not with fire, but with a kind of dark hilarity only trauma survivors truly understand. 2nd June 2013 was one of those days.

I wrote this in my diary after yet another hospital visit, where a well-meaning but infuriating doctor asked me what I believe is the most loaded question in medical history: **"So how are we feeling?"**

Now, I understand it's standard protocol. It's meant to open the conversation gently. But I'd been through hell – slow-burning hell, the kind with delayed diagnoses, surgical chaos, and a cocktail of chemical warfare dressed up in sterile white bags. So on that day, instead of nodding politely or choking back tears, I let sarcasm take the wheel.

Here's what I wrote:

Dear Diary – 2nd June 2013

Note to Self........ALWAYS remember that the highly trained Hospital Emergency Doctors are working from specially designed cue cards that are designed to evoke pure sarcasm from patients!

Question: "So how are we feeling?"

Answer: "Well...apart from being misdiagnosed with dermatitis for 3 years, being told I had Stage 3 breast cancer on Valentine's Day, having both my tits cut off, half my tummy transplanted into my chest and multiple side effects caused by something akin to weed killer being pumped through my veins every 21 days, WE are feeling fine....How 'bout you?"

I don't regret writing that. In fact, I treasure it. It reminds me that even in the bleakest moments, humour was a lifeline. I wasn't okay – but I could still find the absurdity, still reclaim a little power in the way I told my story – even if only to myself.

That's the thing about surviving: it's not always graceful. Sometimes it's messy, sarcastic, and written in block capitals with a biro while wearing a paper gown – open at the back.

Contents

PART ONE

Breathe First: Orientation & Reflections

Dear Reader

For You

If you’ve ever sat across from a doctor and felt unsure how to begin - or walked away wishing you’d said more, remembered more, or been truly heard - you’re not alone.

Over the years, I’ve met so many thoughtful, articulate people who suddenly go quiet in clinical settings. The pressure, the pace, the unfamiliar language - it can make even the clearest voice feel like it’s caught in fog.

That’s why ***Hey Doc, This Is My Story*** doesn’t try to capture everything at once. It’s not a medical file. It’s not a symptom tracker with fifty tabs. It’s something gentler - more human, more you.

Think of this journal like a pocket lantern - small, steady, and designed to light the path just ahead. It’s a quiet companion to help you gather your thoughts, record what matters, and share what’s most important in your own way, in your own time.

This journal is for real people with real stories - not just diagnoses, but lives.

Whether you're navigating a new condition, seeking better care, or simply want a clearer voice in your own wellness journey, these pages are here for you.

Start where you are. Write what you know. Add more as you go. Even just a few words can change everything.

With warmth, courage, and a listening heart,

Hope Fields

Welcome To Your Story

The Appointment Was in Ten Minutes - and I Couldn't Remember Which Doctor I Was Seeing

I still remember the metallic taste of panic that morning. I'd parked outside the oncology clinic, flipped through the contacts on my iPhone, and realized - again - that I wasn't sure which specialist I was about to meet. Was it Dr Lee, my radiation oncologist, with the warm laugh? Or Dr Nguyen, the quiet genius who managed my bone scans? Until cancer, my phone held family birthdays, recipes, and travel photos - anything but physician numbers. By the end of treatment, I had seventeen doctors' names, phone numbers, and appointment notes crowding those tiny digital squares.

Somewhere between chemotherapy cycles, radiation burns, and the daily chaos of simply staying alive, I began scribbling everything - symptoms, medication questions, even the jokes that helped me smile - into an ordinary spiral notebook. My shaky handwriting filled every margin, arrow, and asterisk, racing to keep up with my mind.

That notebook became my lifeline. It helped me:

- **Track subtle changes** my doctors needed to hear.
- **Spot patterns** in side effects before they spiraled.
- **Jot questions** the moment they popped into my head - because chemo brain doesn't wait politely until office hours.
- **Hand over clear snapshots** of my story to whichever specialist appeared next (sometimes one I hadn't expected).

Over time, the notebook's messy scrawl morphed into structure: headings, check-boxes, little "Remember this!" flags. Friends going through their own diagnoses asked for copies. Nurses photocopied pages. A palliative-care doctor told me, "I wish every patient had something like this. It would save so much heartache."

That seed grew into the book you're holding: **Hey Doc. This Is My Story** - a guided journal designed to keep your health story in one compassionate, portable place.

Why a Guided Journal - Not Just Another "Fill-in-the-Blanks" Notebook?

Low-content journals offer empty lines; you deserve more. Fighting illness (be it cancer, chronic pain, autoimmune challenges, or the mental-health storms that often follow) is a full-body sport. You need prompts that:

- **Nudge you toward the details clinicians crave**

- med changes, symptom timelines, lab results - in a format that actually makes sense when you're exhausted.

- **Invite honest reflection, fear, and hope** because data without emotion is only half the picture.
- **Keep caregivers in the loop** - partners, adult children, friends - so you don't have to retell the same story when you're running on fumes.
- **Celebrate tiny victories** along the way: the first full meal after surgery, the afternoon you walked to the mailbox without needing a nap (trust me, it's a thing), the laugh that burst out of nowhere.

Who Will Benefit

- **Patients navigating new or long-term diagnoses** - from oncology to endocrinology.
- **Caregivers** juggling appointment calendars, medication lists, and the unspoken fear of missing something vital.
- **Medical teams** are grateful for concise histories and clear questions (they truly do cheer when a patient is prepared).
- **Anyone living with "hidden" conditions** - mental-health warriors, chronic-pain survivors, autoimmune explorers - who often struggle to prove that what hurts can't always be seen.

What You'll Find Inside

- **A Warm Welcome & How-to-Use Guide** – quick enough to read in a waiting room, thorough sufficient to set you up for success.
- **Gather Your Story** – prompts for diagnosis history, symptom trackers, medication overviews, emergency contacts, and "Hospital Go-Bag" checklists.
- **The Appointment Companion** – question builders, note pages framed for follow-up actions, and a simple rating scale so doctors can gauge what matters most today.
- **Reflections & Resilience** – space for feelings, faith, humor, and those random 3 a.m. thoughts that deserve daylight.
- **Sticky Note-to-Self Moments** – encouraging reminders in the margins because healing is not only clinical; it's profoundly human.

A Quick Word of Encouragement

If flipping through these pages feels daunting, remember: you don't have to complete everything tonight. Start with your next appointment date or with the one question that keeps echoing in your mind. This journal is here to lighten – not add to – the load.

You're not just a checklist of vitals; you're a living, breathing story. Your feelings, your fears, your hard-won knowledge - they all matter. The more clearly you can share that story, the better your team can help you write the following healthier chapter. And you deserve a chapter that honors everything you've endured and everything you're still becoming.

From one survivor – and seventeen doctors' phone numbers – to you: let's make sure your story never gets lost in the shuffle again. Open to page one, take a deep breath, and say it with me:

"Hey Doc, this is my story."

How To Use This Journal

There is No Wrong Way

THIS IS YOUR SPACE - your story, your scribbles, your small victories, and even your messy middle parts.

Whether you're navigating a new diagnosis or chronic condition, supporting a loved one, or trying to make sense of test results and tangled emotions, this journal is here to help you gather what matters and let go of what doesn't.

Start with breath, not pressure.

Begin with the breathing page or simply flip to a section that feels most useful today. You don’t have to fill in every box or complete it in order.

Tell your story, your way

Use the "This Is My Story" section to share the big picture - your diagnosis, timeline, or simply what life feels like right now. This becomes a helpful summary for doctors and a moment of validation for you.

Prepare before appointments

Flip to the appointment prep pages and jot down questions, symptoms, or concerns while they're fresh. These pages are structured to help you walk into appointments feeling organized—even on hard days.

Track what your body's trying to say

Use the symptom tracker and test sections to spot patterns, side effects, or changes that matter. These notes help your medical team make better decisions - and help you feel more in control.

Leave room for feelings

The reflections and future self pages aren't just extras - they're medicine of another kind. Whether you write a little or a lot, your emotional story deserves space too.

Stick notes where they matter

Look out for the Sticky Note-to-Self reminders and encouragements in the margins. These aren't just cute - they're anchors for days when you forget how far you've come.

Customize as you go

Add your own tabs, color in the borders, tape in appointment cards or letters. This is your brave book - make it feel like you.

Final Thought

Some days, all you'll write is the date. Other days, your pen won't stop.

Both are valid.

This journal isn't just about tracking symptoms - it's about witnessing your story with compassion.

One page at a time...

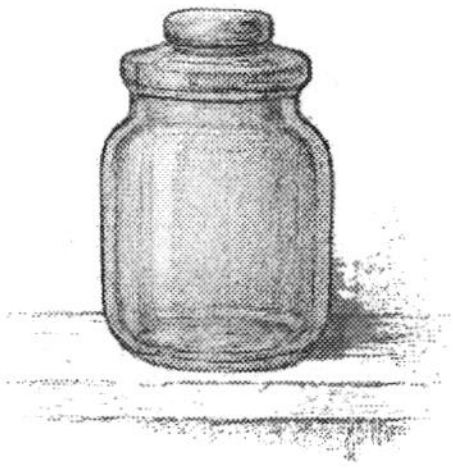

The Jar That Listened

A Short Story

LET ME TELL YOU a story... Not the loud kind, with dragons or battles or shiny trophies – but a quiet one. The kind that might be whispered when the lights are low. The kind that stays with you, long after the telling.

There was once a jar. Not a fancy jar – no gold trim, no glowing stones. Just a simple jar with a smooth glass belly and a lid that didn't squeak. It sat on a shelf for a long time. Waiting. Listening...

No one knew exactly where it came from.

Some said it was given. Some said it just appeared one day – when someone needed it most.

What made the jar special wasn't how it looked.

It was what it did. You see, when people didn't know what to say – when their thoughts felt too tangled, or their pain didn't have words, they would sit quietly with the jar.

And sometimes, just sometimes, they would lean close and whisper.

Not full sentences. Sometimes just a sigh. A memory. A fear that had never been spoken aloud.

And the jar? It never interrupted. Never corrected. Never asked for more than was given. It just listened. And somehow, that was enough.

Over time, people began to write their whispers down - folded them into tiny notes, and tucked them beneath the lid. Not to be fixed. Not to be judged. Just to be held.

The jar didn't solve things. But it softened the sharp edges.

And for those who had never felt heard, it became a beginning.

This journal... well, it's a bit like that jar. You don't have to explain everything. You don't have to make it perfect. You just have to begin.

Whatever you need to whisper – you can put it here.

Breathing Exercises

How To Use This Breathing Page

A soft place to land when everything feels a little too much.

Before you dive into the rest of this book, pause here.

This page is your gentle invitation to exhale - fully and without apology.

Whether your heart is racing, your thoughts are tangling, or your body feels tense, this moment is for you.

Let's breathe together.

Breathing Exercise 1:

The 4-7-8 Calm Down

A quiet rhythm to soothe the nervous system.

Breathe in through your nose for 4 seconds

Hold that breath gently for 7 seconds

Exhale slowly through your mouth for 8 seconds

Repeat 4 times (Or as many as you need - no rush.)

Tip: Imagine blowing out a candle on your exhale - slow and steady.

Breathing Exercise 2:

Bubble Belly Breathing

A soft belly, a softer mind.

Place one hand on your belly and one on your chest.

Breathe in deeply through your nose.

Feel your belly rise like a balloon.

Breathe out through your mouth.

Feel your belly fall like the tide going out.

Repeat 5 times, watching your hands gently move with each breath.

You're safe to slow down.

Breathing Exercise 3:

Feather Breath (Visual Aid Optional)

Imagine holding a delicate feather in front of you.

Breathe in slowly...

Now exhale as if trying not to blow the feather away.

Soft. Gentle. Controlled.

Repeat until your body feels a little looser, and your thoughts feel a little kinder.

Gentle Note to the Reader

Your breath is always with you - a quiet companion, even when words fail.

You don't need to fix everything.

You just need to breathe through this one moment.

Go Gently

Expression Pages

This Is Your Space

There are some thoughts that can't be written in straight lines. Some feelings that live better in swirls, colors, or quiet marks on a page.

These pages are just for you – to draw, doodle, scribble, sketch, or simply rest. No rules, no pressure. Just a little room to breathe, in whatever way you need.

Go gently. You're doing better than you think.

QUICK START GUIDE

Start Here – You're Not Alone

SOMETIMES YOU DON'T NEED to begin at the beginning. You just need the *right page for right now*.

Feeling anxious or overwhelmed?

Turn to the "Breathe First" pages (Part One – *Orientation & Reflections*)
Let your breath guide you before anything else.

Preparing for an appointment?

Flip to "Before My Next Appointment" (Page 37)
A gentle space to help you get clear, calm, and ready.

Not sure what to say or where to start?

Try "Unfiltered Thoughts – WARTS & All" (Page 22)
Sometimes the messiest thoughts are the most important.

Need a break?

Use a "Go Gently – Expression Page"

There's space to doodle, scribble, or simply be still.

Let this book meet you where you are.
You don't have to fill it all at once.
You don't even have to fill it in order.

Your story. Your pace. Your way.

PART TWO

Your Story: Naming What Matters

This Is My Story

Guided Questions

EVERYONE HAS A BEGINNING. Sometimes it's clear and sharp, like a memory etched in stone. Sometimes it's soft and hard to find.

Wherever your story begins, this space is for you.

Use it to remember, to reflect, or to simply notice what has brought you here.

1. What was happening in your life when things first changed?

2. How did you first know something was wrong – or different?

3. What moments feel important to remember?

4. Is there a piece of the story no one else knows?

Living With This

Guided Questions

THIS PART OF YOUR story is still unfolding. It might look different every day. And that's okay.

This space is for naming what it's like to live with what you're carrying – physically, emotionally, or otherwise.

What does a typical day look like right now?

What are the hardest parts?

What helps?

What do you wish people understood about your experience?

For Future Me

Guided Questions

THIS IS YOUR SPACE for hope.

Whether you whisper a wish, set an intention, or leave a message for your future self – these pages are a gentle way to speak to the road ahead.

What do I want to remember when things feel hard?

What do I hope for myself?

What might future me need to hear?

A letter to myself:

Dear Me...

PART THREE

The Inner Landscape: Emotions & Reflections

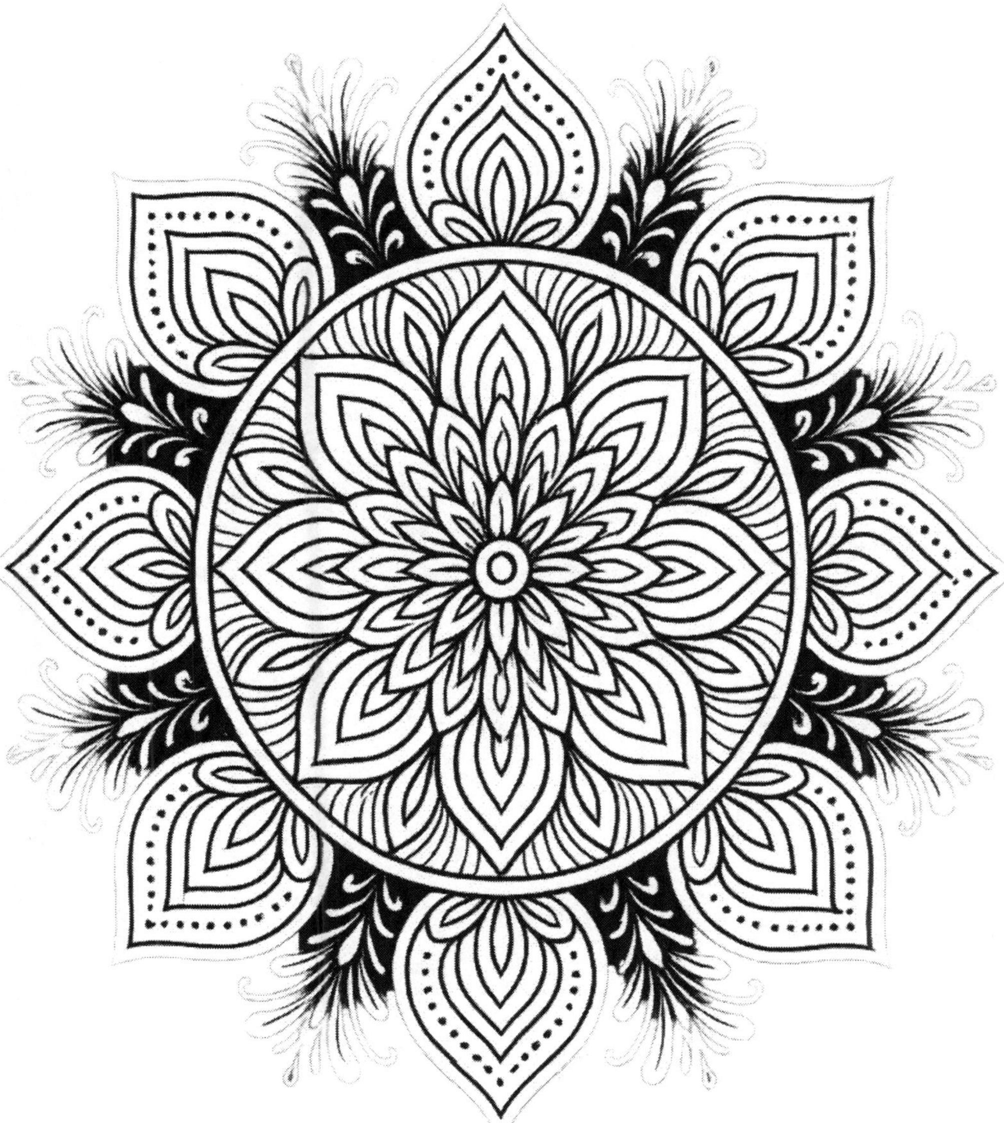

Moonlight Pages

For What Can't Be Said

SOME THOUGHTS HIDE IN the shadows.
Others come out only when things are soft and still, like the hush of moonlight on a windowsill.

Use these pages however you like – for what you feel, what you fear, or what you haven't found the words for yet.

Let the quiet do the talking.

Still Space

Just For You

Sometimes the world is loud.
These pages are here for the quiet things: the little moments, the not-quite-words, the shapes your feelings make when they're left alone for a while.

Draw. Scribble. Breathe.

This is still your story, even when you're not sure what to say.

Unfiltered Thoughts

WARTS & All!

Let's be real for a moment.

NOT EVERY THOUGHT WE have is graceful, wise, or even kind. Some are tangled, loud, messy. Others hide in quiet corners, waiting for us to notice them. And some – well, they're just plain weird.

But they're all part of *you*.

This space isn't for tidy answers or fixed-up feelings. It's for raw honesty. The kind you whisper into your pillow or think about in waiting rooms. It's where you can dump the junk drawer of your mind and not worry about spelling, grammar, or what anyone might think. No need to explain or make sense of it. Just get it out.

This is where the healing often begins – in the messy middle, not the perfect end.

So go on. Be unfiltered. Be real. WARTS & all.

You Are Brave!

The Poem

If you've filled just one page, you've begun.

If you've poured your heart out across many, you've made space for healing.

And if you've skipped around, doodled in the margins, or whispered truths between the lines –
you've used this journal exactly as it was meant to be used.

Your story is valid.
Your words matter.
You are not alone.

May this book remind you that what's inside you deserves to be heard -
even when it's complicated, even when it's unfinished,
even when no one else quite understands.

You've taken the brave step of writing it down.

And that is enough because...

This Is Your Brave Book!

Growing Room

For What Comes Next

HEALING ISN'T ALWAYS TIDY. It's not a straight line or a single moment.
But it *does* make space.

These pages are here for new roots, small beginnings, or dreams that haven't spoken up yet.

There's no right way to grow. Just this moment. This page. And you.

PART FOUR

Support Map: Communication & Next Steps

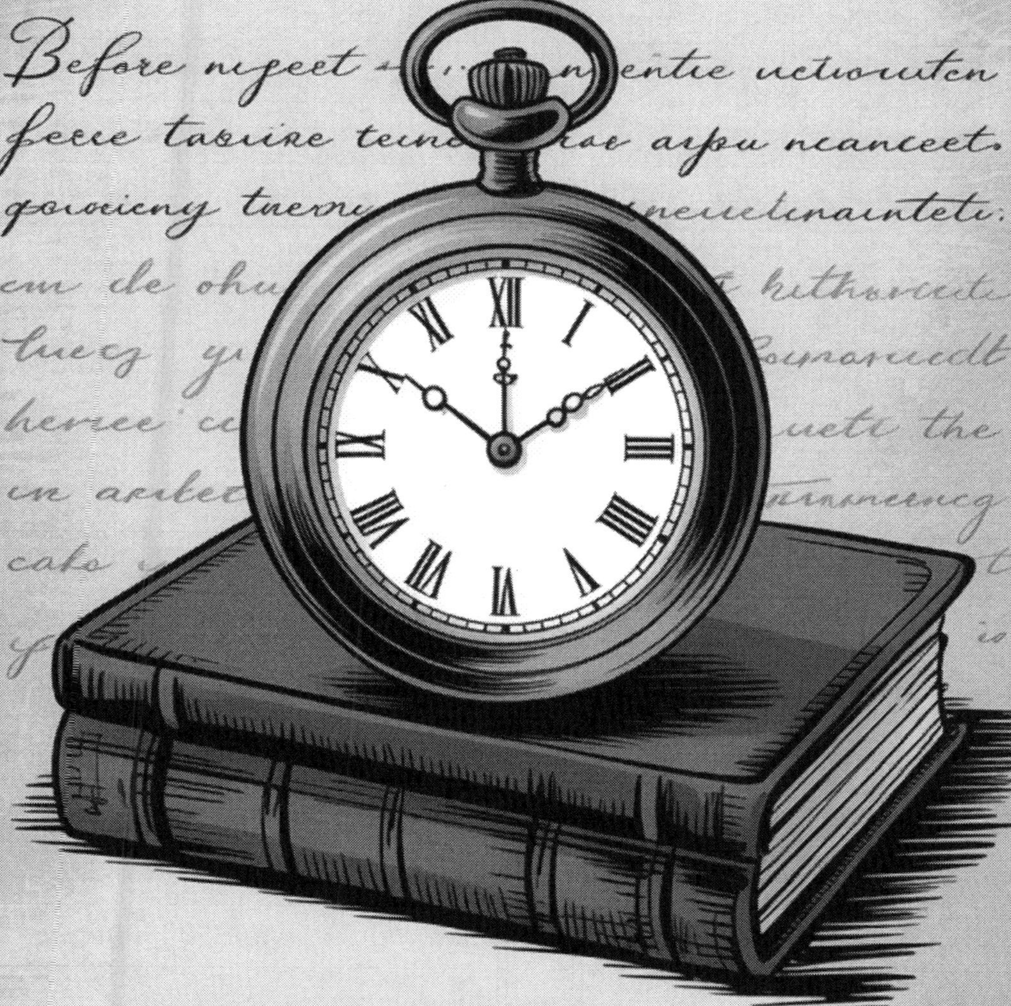

Before my next Appointment

"You can photocopy these pages or use them multiple times"

Before My Next Appt With

____

(Doctor/Specialist/Health Professional's Name)

APPOINYMENT: ______ AM/PM / ___ / ___ / 20_____

Clinic/Hospital/Location:

____

1. What's changed since my last visit?

____

____

2. What concerns do I want to talk about?

3. What questions do I want to ask?

4. What do I hope to get from this appointment?

5. Is there anything I need to bring or prepare?

Appointments can move quickly – this page helps you slow things down before you walk in.

Things I Want to Ask:

Things I Want to Say (But Might Forget):

Symptoms/Changes Since My Last Visit:

Medications, Treatments, or Supplements I've Started/Stopped:

__ Started / Stopped

____

__ Started / Stopped

____

__ Started / Stopped

____

__ Started / Stopped

____

__ Started / Stopped

____

__ Started / Stopped

____

__ Started / Stopped

____

__ Started / Stopped

____

__ Started / Stopped

____

What Matters Most to Me Right Now:

(This could be a concern, a goal, or just something that's been on your heart.)

"Between now and then, I'll give myself grace, gather my thoughts, and remember that even small steps matter"

Test Procedures

You Can Do It

A PLACE TO UNPACK what's happening to your body – and how it feels inside your mind.

You can photocopy these pages or use them multiple times.

BEFORE THE TEST

What is this test or procedure for?
(e.g., to confirm a diagnosis, check on progress, rule something out)

What do I already know about it?
(Write any info you've been told or researched.)

What questions do I still have?
(What would I like to ask my doctor or support team?)

What am I feeling in my body right now as I think about this test?
(Any tension, fear, numbness, hope?)

What do I need to feel more prepared?
(A support person? Clearer information? Something comforting?)

DURING OR JUST AFTER

How did the procedure or test go?
(Write what happened as clearly or vaguely as feels right.)

Did anything surprise me?
(Emotionally, physically, or practically.)

Who helped me feel safe or calm?
(Write their name or describe them if you'd like.)

What do I want to remember about this experience—just for me?
(Any insight, strength, or even frustration worth noting.)

WAITING FOR RESULTS

What is this waiting period like for me?
(Am I feeling calm, distracted, worried?)

What helps me pass the time gently?
(Is there something I can do today that feels grounding?)

What do I need to hear from others right now?
(Support, space, distraction?)

Is there anything I'd like to say to my future self—no matter what the results show?
(Encouragement, kindness, truth.)

Before My Next Appt With

____

(Doctor/Specialist/Health Professional's Name)

APPOINYMENT: ______ AM/PM / ___ / ___ / 20_____

Clinic/Hospital/Location:

____

1. What's changed since my last visit?

____

____

2. What concerns do I want to talk about?

____

____

3. What questions do I want to ask?

4. What do I hope to get from this appointment?

5. Is there anything I need to bring or prepare?

Appointments can move quickly – this page helps you slow things down before you walk in.

Things I Want to Ask:

Things I Want to Say (But Might Forget):

Symptoms/Changes Since My Last Visit:

Medications, Treatments, or Supplements I've Started/Stopped:

__ Started / Stopped

____

__ Started / Stopped

__ Started / Stopped

__ Started / Stopped

__ Started / Stopped

__ Started / Stopped

__ Started / Stopped

__ Started / Stopped

__ Started / Stopped

What Matters Most to Me Right Now:

(This could be a concern, a goal, or just something that's been on your heart.)

"Between now and then, I'll give myself grace, gather my thoughts, and remember that even small steps matter"

Before My Next Appt With

____

(Doctor/Specialist/Health Professional's Name)

APPOINYMENT: ______ AM/PM / ___ / ___ / 20_____

Clinic/Hospital/Location:

____

1. What's changed since my last visit?

____

____

2. What concerns do I want to talk about?

____

____

3. What questions do I want to ask?

4. What do I hope to get from this appointment?

5. Is there anything I need to bring or prepare?

Appointments can move quickly – this page helps you slow things down before you walk in.

Things I Want to Ask:

Things I Want to Say (But Might Forget):

Symptoms/Changes Since My Last Visit:

Medications, Treatments, or Supplements I've Started/Stopped:

__ Started / Stopped

__ Started / Stopped

__ Started / Stopped

__ Started / Stopped

__ Started / Stopped

__ Started / Stopped

__ Started / Stopped

__ Started / Stopped

__ Started / Stopped

What Matters Most to Me Right Now:

(This could be a concern, a goal, or just something that's been on your heart.)

"Between now and then, I'll give myself grace, gather my thoughts, and remember that even small steps matter"

Symptom & Trigger Tracker Page...

Use this page to note symptoms as they arise, and gently reflect on what may have contributed. You don't need to know everything - just jot down what you notice. Over time, patterns may appear that help you understand and better support your body.

Date Used: ____/____/______

Symptom (e.g., Fatigue, Pain, Brain Fog): ______________________________

____

____

ntensity: 1-5)_____ Duration: __________ (Approx min/hrs/days)

Possible Triggers? ____

____

(Stress, food, hormones, weather, sleep, emotions etc.)

What Happened? ____

(Any remedy, habit, or rest that brought relief)

____

Notes/Reflections: (Emotional response or observations) ______________

____

____

____

____

____

Medical Snapshot Page...

A calm, one-page summary of the most important information to help tell your story.

This page is here to support you when you're too tired, stressed, or overwhelmed to remember every detail. Think of it as your backup voice - clear, kind, and right at your fingertips.

Herb Name: ____

Date Used: _____/_____/______

Preparation Method (e.g., Tea, Salve, Tincture): ________________

____

____

____

Why Did I Use It? ____________________________________

____

How Did It Make Me Feel? ______________________________

____

Any Side Effects & Reactions? ___________________________

____

____

Would I Use It Again? _________________________________

Notes & Observations: _________________________________

____

____

____

After Care & Next Steps

Guided Questions

WHAT NEW DECISIONS DO I need to make?

Who do I want to talk to next?

What have I learned from this experience?

What would I tell someone else going through this?

Closing Thoughts

From One Story to Another…

You've done something remarkable.

WHETHER YOU FILLED EVERY page or simply sat with a few, you showed up for yourself in a way that matters. You paused. You reflected. You told the truth – even when it was messy, complicated, or uncertain.

That takes courage.

This journal was never about having the perfect words. It was always about making space for the real ones – the tired ones, the tender ones, the honest ones. The ones that too often go unheard in crowded waiting rooms or rushed appointments.

So wherever you go from here – whatever pages remain blank or scribbled or stained with tears – please remember:

Your story matters.
Your questions are valid.
Your voice is worth hearing.

And you are not alone.

With deep respect and a listening heart,
Hope Fields

My Reflection Journal

Make a Difference with Your Review

Ulock the Power of Generosity

"Every time we tell the truth of our own journey, we give someone else permission to begin theirs." – Natalie Mills

A Little Note Before You Close the Cover...

Your Turn to Inspire Someone Else's Reset

Have you ever hit a season of life that felt like a plot twist – midlife changes, new questions, an itch for something more – and wondered if anyone else really gets it? That's exactly why *Mindful Midlife Reset* was written: to give every woman permission to pause, listen, and shape her next chapter with courage (and a healthy dash of humor).

Now you can help the next reader who's standing right where you once stood – curious, maybe a little restless, and ready for a gentle nudge.

Why your review matters

By sharing a few honest sentences, you can help another woman:

Realize she's not alone in the messy, beautiful middle years

Discover simple tools for calm, clarity, and self-kindness

Feel brave enough to rewrite her own story – one mindful step at a time

It only takes a minute

Pop over to the review section where you found this book and jot a few genuine words:

What resonated most for you?

Which practice or story lit a spark?

Why would you recommend this book to someone navigating midlife?

OR use this link:
[https://www.amazon.com/review/review-your-purchases/?asin= 1923524062]

Hit **Submit** and know you've just left a trail of encouragement – like a warm cup of tea waiting for the next traveler.

Thank you, from the bottom of my midlife-mischief-loving heart, for helping other women discover their own fresh start.

With gratitude,
Natalie Mills
Author of *Mindful Midlife Reset*

References

1. Weil, A. (n.d.). *Breathing: Three exercises*. Dr. Weil. Retrieved from https://www.drweil.com/health-wellness/body-mind-spirit/stress-anxiety/breathing-three-exercises/

2. Ma, X., Yue, Z. Q., Gong, Z. Q., Zhang, H., Duan, N. Y., Shi, Y. T., Wei, G. X., & Li, Y. F. (2017). The effect of diaphragmatic breathing on attention, negative affect, and stress in healthy adults. *Frontiers in Psychology, 8*, 874. https://doi.org/10.3389/fpsyg.2017.00874

3. Khoury, B., Sharma, M., Rush, S. E., & Fournier, C. (2015). Mindfulness-based stress reduction for healthy individuals: A meta-analysis. *Journal of Psychosomatic Research, 78*(6), 519–528. https://doi.org/10.1016/j.jpsychores.2015.03.009

4. Boer, K. A. (2025). *Chemo sunrise: A poetic & picturesque journey.* 1957 Publishing

Notes on Sources

The reflections, prompts, and exercises in this journal were created by the author and informed by her personal experience, holistic practice, and conversations with medical professionals over time.

This guided journal does not offer medical advice and is not intended to diagnose or treat any condition. For all health matters, please consult with your qualified care provider.

Note: Some reflections and narrative content in this journal were published initially in *Chemo Sunrise: A Poetic & Picturesque Journey* by Kerry Anne Boer (2025). These have been adapted here with the author's full permission and intention to support broader conversations about healing.

Made in the USA
Monee, IL
11 November 2026

cb3bbaf2-c5df-4103-976f-491bd2a873abR02